Tesamorelin

The Skeptic's Guide: How to Evaluate Claims, Evidence, and Trade-offs Without Guesswork

mf

Disclaimer

By reading this guide, you are accepting the terms of this disclaimer in full. If you do not agree with these terms, please do not read or use this guide.

All content within this guide is provided for informational and educational purposes only and should not be considered medical, psychological, or other professional advice. The author is not a doctor, physician, psychologist, psychotherapist, counselor, or licensed healthcare provider. Reading or using this guide does not establish any form of a patient-client or therapeutic relationship.

Always consult with a physician, licensed therapist, or other qualified health professional regarding any questions or concerns you may have about your physical or mental health. Never disregard professional advice or delay seeking it because of something you have read in this guide.

The information presented in this guide is based on general research, personal interpretation, and publicly available sources. While reasonable efforts have been made to provide accurate and current information, the author and publisher make no representations or warranties about the completeness, accuracy, reliability, or suitability of the content. The author and publisher shall not be held liable for any errors, omissions, or outcomes related to the use of this guide.

You acknowledge that you are solely responsible for how you choose to use the information in this guide and that any actions you take based on this content are undertaken at your own risk. The publisher shall not be liable for any loss, injury, or damages arising from the application of any information provided herein.

This guide does not promise or guarantee any specific result, outcome, or improvement in well-being, mental health, or nervous system regulation. Individual results may vary.

Where applicable, any tools, concepts, or names mentioned are the property of their respective owners and are used strictly for identification or illustrative purposes. Their mention does not imply endorsement. Any individuals shown in the cover or promotional images are stock photography models, and image rights have been obtained through appropriate licensing agreements.

Table of Contents

Introduction

If you have started researching Tesamorelin, you have likely found yourself lost in a thicket of overlapping claims about its benefits, risks, and intended uses. Information presented online, in forums, and even in some medical settings frequently conflicts, some sources touting Tesamorelin as a breakthrough for fat reduction and metabolic health, others warning of potential adverse effects, and still others positioning it as a panacea for a range of off-label applications. As a skeptic, your challenge is to sort through these competing claims and make sense of what is actually supported by robust evidence, what is speculative, and what might be outright misinformation.

The consequences of acting on poorly evidenced or incomplete Tesamorelin information are far from trivial. Within medical practice, basing decisions on unproven claims can expose patients to unnecessary risks or withhold legitimate treatments that have been shown to work. In wellness and consumer spaces, reliance on hype or anecdotal testimonies can lead to costly, ineffective, or potentially harmful self-experimentation.

For a medication like Tesamorelin, which is approved for specific indications such as reducing excess abdominal fat in HIV-infected patients with lipodystrophy, misunderstanding its profile can impact health, safety, and trust in evidence-based practices.

Inconsistent messaging about Tesamorelin's safety and efficacy often stems from cherry-picked data, anecdotal outcomes, misinterpretation of complex medical studies, or a lack of clarity on how long results take to appear. For instance, while some users expect rapid effects from Tesamorelin, the clinical evidence suggests a timeline for visible results that spans several weeks and depends on ongoing administration.

Additionally, side effects can range from mild to significant, and a clear, evidence-based understanding is essential before deciding whether the benefits outweigh the risks in any specific scenario.

This guide is built for those seeking clarity without hype. Here, you'll gain practical tools that make it possible to evaluate Tesamorelin claims with confidence rather than guesswork. You will learn how to identify which claims have legitimate backing, especially ones confirmed through large clinical trials or regulatory review versus those supported merely by anecdote or low-quality reports.

We'll break down how to classify supporting evidence by tier, whether it comes from preclinical models, controlled human trials, or postmarketing surveillance data. Understanding these distinctions is fundamental for making informed choices and recognizing where the uncertainties still lie.

You will also discover frameworks for recognizing and weighing the nuanced trade-offs around Tesamorelin use. This includes how to construct simple yet powerful comparison tables, apply stepwise risk assessments, and trace the origins of popular claims through both marketing and peer-reviewed literature. Practical guidance will help you recognize frequent misinterpretations like confusing statistically significant changes for clinically meaningful ones, or overgeneralizing limited study results as well as avoid common decision-making pitfalls.

This guide is not a substitute for individualized medical advice; you should always consult a qualified healthcare provider for clinical decisions. Nor will you find in-depth biochemistry, gray-market sourcing, or illicit use strategies in these pages. Our focus will remain tightly on transparent evaluation, ethical use, and science-backed information relevant to approved and investigational contexts for Tesamorelin.

By the end of this guide, you will know how to:

- Identify and vet valid Tesamorelin claims

- Classify evidence to distinguish between robust and weak support
- Systematically assess risk–benefit trade-offs
- Build comparison tables for claims and alternatives
- Apply structured risk frameworks to decision-making
- Sample recipes of kimchi dishes Recognize and correct for common misinterpretations of Tesamorelin data

With these tools, you'll be equipped to navigate the world of Tesamorelin information, evaluate new claims as they arise, and act with both skepticism and confidence in your knowledge.

Tesamorelin Fundamentals Checklist

For anyone approaching Tesamorelin with a skeptic's mindset, the first step is building a grounded understanding of exactly what the compound is and what it is not. This means not only knowing the official definition, uses, and approved frameworks that govern it, but also being precise about how Tesamorelin fits among related peptides, how regulations limit access, and what specific contraindications matter for any evidence-based evaluation.

What follows is a comprehensive checklist that will enable you to systematically vet claims about Tesamorelin's function, status, and suitability, arming you with facts before stepping into more complex analyses.

Defining Tesamorelin: Approved Indications, Mechanism, and Nature

Tesamorelin is best understood as a synthetic analog of growth hormone–releasing hormone (GHRH). Its design closely mimics the structure of naturally occurring GHRH, allowing it to bind to its corresponding receptors on the pituitary gland. This action stimulates the release of endogenous growth hormone, which in turn can affect fat metabolism, among other physiological processes.

On an approval basis, Tesamorelin is not a general growth hormone therapy or an anti-aging peptide. It has received specific regulatory endorsement for reducing excess abdominal fat technically called visceral adipose tissue in HIV-infected patients with lipodystrophy.

This population experiences abnormal fat distribution due, in part, to long-term antiretroviral therapy, affecting both health outcomes and quality of life. Its mechanism stems directly from its GHRH analog profile. Tesamorelin triggers the pituitary to produce and secrete increased growth hormone; however, it does not act as growth hormone itself.

Checklist Summary:

- Is Tesamorelin a synthetic compound or naturally derived? Synthetic GHRH analog.
- What is the approved medical use? Reduction of excess abdominal fat in HIV-infected patients with lipodystrophy.
- What is its core mechanism? Binds to pituitary GHRH receptors, stimulating endogenous growth hormone release.

- Does it have growth hormones like effects directly? No; it acts only by stimulating the body's own GH production.

A clear grasp of these facts dispels multiple common misconceptions often encountered in wellness circles, such as the notion that Tesamorelin is simply another form of growth hormone or an "anti-aging" shot. Evaluating any further claim therapeutic or adverse must be done within this mechanistic and regulatory context.

Approved Uses and Main Investigational Directions

A decisive feature of Tesamorelin's status is the distinction between what it is approved to treat, what it is studied for, and what is merely hypothesized. Skeptics should insist on separating sanctioned therapeutic roles from off-label, experimental, or anecdotal uses. Here is a structured summary to organize this understanding:

Currently Approved Use:

Reduction of visceral adipose tissue in HIV-infected adults diagnosed with lipodystrophy (especially those who experience harmful or distressing fat accumulation in the abdomen due to HIV therapy).

Key Points About Approved Use:

- Tesamorelin is indicated solely for adult patients; it is not approved for use in children or adolescents.
- Its use is targeted; regulatory approval does not extend to general obesity or non-HIV-related fat accumulation.
- The clinical efficacy is defined in terms of measurable reductions in visceral fat, typically seen over a span of several weeks of continuous administration.

Main Investigational Directions:

- While the guide's remit is limited to evidence-backed evaluation, notable investigational directions have involved examining Tesamorelin's effects on metabolic health, cognitive function, and even its use as an adjunct in non-HIV populations. However, these directions remain investigational and are not part of official approved indications.
- Claims regarding "anti-aging" benefits or off-label enhancement often lack robust, large-scale clinical evidence and should be distinguished from regulated, studied uses.

Regulatory and Prescription Status Framework by Jurisdiction

Understanding where Tesamorelin fits within the legal and regulatory landscapes is essential for two reasons. First, it sets boundaries around what is permitted in medical settings. Second, it highlights where pseudo-medical or gray-market activity may color perceptions and the dissemination of information.

Prescription Status Overview:

- In most jurisdictions, including the United States and Canada, Tesamorelin is a prescription-only medication authorized under tightly controlled conditions.
- It is classified and dispensed under trade names (notably Egrifta), and is available only by prescription after a qualifying diagnosis typically HIV-associated lipodystrophy.
- Prescribers are usually required to document the specific clinical condition and to comply with monitoring and follow-up requirements dictated by national and regional medical authorities.
- In countries or contexts where Tesamorelin is not formally approved, it is either inaccessible legally or, when acquired through unregulated channels, carries significant risk—both for health and legal outcomes.

Jurisdictional Framework Checklist:

- Is Tesamorelin approved for use in general obesity? No; only for HIV patients with lipodystrophy.
- Can it be obtained over the counter or online without a prescription? Not legally in most countries.

- Are there mandatory monitoring or documentation requirements? Yes; typically required for each prescribed use.
- Is off-label marketing or promotion permitted? No; marketing is restricted to approved indications and regulated by enforcement agencies.

These regulatory boundaries are not simply bureaucratic hurdles. They reflect the limits of substantiated benefit and the actual evidence reviewed by regulatory agencies. If a claim about Tesamorelin's availability, use, or risk profile appears to disregard these constraints, it may signal misinformation or gray-zone marketing activity.

Summary Chart of Essential Contraindications and Restrictions

A crucial aspect of the fundamentals checklist is recognizing when Tesamorelin is clearly contraindicated or should only be prescribed under the most careful circumstances.

Major Contraindications:

- ***Hypersensitivity to Tesamorelin or any formulation component***: Patients with documented allergies to the active peptide or excipients should not use Tesamorelin.
- ***Known or suspected pregnancy***: Tesamorelin should not be used during pregnancy, as sufficient safety data

do not exist and GH pathway modulation could potentially affect fetal development.

- ***Active malignancy***: Because Tesamorelin stimulates the growth hormone axis, it is contraindicated in patients with known or suspected active malignancy. This is based on the potential for growth-promoting effects on neoplastic tissue.
- ***Pituitary tumors or surgery***: Increased GH levels can exacerbate pituitary abnormalities or interfere with healing in post-surgical states.

Relative Restrictions and Cautions:

- Individuals with a history of glucose intolerance or diabetes should use Tesamorelin cautiously, given potential to influence glucose metabolism.
- Its safety and efficacy have not been established in children, so use in pediatric populations is not recommended.

Table 1: Summary Chart

Contraindication	Description and Notes
Allergy/ Hypersensitivity	Documented allergy to Tesamorelin or formulation component
Pregnancy	Should not be used; potential risk to fetus
Active malignancy	Contraindicated; potential to stimulate tumor growth
Pituitary tumor/ surgery	Use only with great caution or not at all
Diabetes/ glucose intolerance	Increased risk for glycemic disturbance monitor closely
Pediatric use	Not established should be avoided

A genuinely skeptical approach involves ensuring any claim about Tesamorelin use is contextualized against these well-established contraindications and restrictions.

Protocol for Differentiating Tesamorelin from Similar Peptides and GH Analogs

One of the greatest sources of confusion even among healthcare professionals is the conflation of Tesamorelin with various other peptides, "growth hormone secretagogues," or direct GH analogs. For evidence-based evaluation, the distinctions matter profoundly, both for interpreting research and for understanding side effect profiles, availability, and expected outcomes.

Key Differentiators:

1. **Structure and Action:**
    - Tesamorelin is a modified segment of human GHRH. It acts at the level of the GHRH receptor on the pituitary, not as growth hormone itself.
    - Direct growth hormone (GH) analogs such as recombinant human growth hormone (rhGH) bypass upstream regulatory feedback loops, leading to different systemic effects and risk profiles.

2. **Indication Specificity:**

   Tesamorelin is approved for a limited indication (HIV-associated lipodystrophy). Most GH analogs have different or broader indications, often in pediatric growth disorders or adult GH deficiency.

3. **Biological Impact Timeline:**

   - The effects of Tesamorelin, including measurable reductions in visceral fat, typically unfold over several weeks of regular administration, as opposed to the rapid and sometimes more pronounced effects of direct GH administration.
   - Differences in onset and magnitude of side effects are also observed, with Tesamorelin's indirect mechanism generally leading to a different safety profile.

4. **Regulation and Monitoring:**

   Both Tesamorelin and GH analogs are strictly regulated, but confusion often arises when non-prescription or "research chemical" versions are marketed for broad anti-aging or bodybuilding purposes not supported by regulatory review or large trials.

Differentiation Protocol:

1. Determine the molecular type (GHRH analog vs direct GH analog vs ghrelin mimetic).
2. Compare approved indications: are they identical or substantially different?
3. Identify the route and time course of action; Tesamorelin produces effects over weeks, not days.
4. Review the regulatory status and approved prescribing framework.
5. Examine potential side effect risks based on mechanism (indirect activation vs direct hormone effect).

Practical Checklist for Differentiation:

- Is the agent a GHRH analog (like Tesamorelin) or a direct substitute for growth hormone?
- Has it been approved for visceral fat reduction in HIV lipodystrophy, or is its main indication different?
- Does the safety and monitoring framework match Tesamorelin's requirements?
- Are advertised benefits (e.g., rapid muscle growth, "anti-aging reversal") consistent with published timelines and mechanisms?

Armed with this checklist, you will have an objective basis for assessing nearly any claim regarding Tesamorelin's actions, status, or appropriateness. The clarity about its mechanism, tightly defined approval for HIV-related lipodystrophy, and concrete contraindications serves as a filter against exaggerated or improperly generalized statements. Remember: skepticism is most productive when rooted in a methodical evaluation of what is known, what is proven, and what is specifically allowed within the boundaries of established evidence and regulation.

As you continue through this guide, these fundamentals will serve as reference points anchoring your ability to weigh complex claims, evaluate new research, and protect yourself from the confusion and hype that often surround Tesamorelin in both clinical practice and public discourse.

Mechanisms and Biological Pathways Map

A skeptic's approach to Tesamorelin begins with understanding not only what this synthetic peptide is, but precisely how it interacts within the body. This chapter maps the main mechanistic pathways underlying Tesamorelin's effects from the instant it is administered to the resulting physiological changes while clarifying where current science draws its boundaries of certainty. By the end, you will be equipped to dissect mechanistic claims, scrutinize the plausibility of purported benefits and risks, and resist both vague explanations and misplaced hype.

Diagram of Tesamorelin's Primary Action on Growth Hormone Releasing Factor (GHRF) Receptors

Tesamorelin is a synthetic peptide designed to mimic the structure of human growth hormone–releasing hormone (GHRH). Its central mechanism begins at the pituitary gland, a small endocrine organ situated at the base of the brain. After subcutaneous injection, Tesamorelin circulates in the bloodstream until it binds to specific GHRH receptors located on the surface of somatotroph cells in the anterior pituitary. This interaction does not involve direct hormone replacement, but instead acts as a biological signal, an external "on switch" that mimics the body's own GHRH activity.

What sets Tesamorelin apart from other compounds is its highly selective binding to these GHRH receptors. When bound, it triggers a cascade resulting in the synthesis and secretion of endogenous growth hormone (GH). The process is tightly regulated and mimics the body's own physiological feedback systems, distinguishing it from the less nuanced effects of direct GH administration.

This specificity lies at the heart of both its therapeutic value and side effect profile: Tesamorelin does not flood the body with exogenous GH, but rather encourages the pituitary to do its natural job, albeit in a targeted and augmented manner.

Stepwise Sequence of Expected Molecular Effects from Administration to Target Tissue Response

The mechanistic journey of Tesamorelin unfolds in several well-documented steps:

1. ***Administration***: Tesamorelin is injected subcutaneously, most often into the abdominal area.

2. ***Systemic Absorption***: Following injection, the peptide enters systemic circulation, avoiding breakdown in the gastrointestinal tract.
3. ***Receptor Binding***: Tesamorelin travels to the anterior pituitary gland, where it binds selectively to GHRH receptors on somatotroph cells.
4. ***Intracellular Signaling***: The binding event activates intracellular signaling pathways particularly cyclic adenosine monophosphate (cAMP) pathways stimulating both synthesis and pulsatile secretion of growth hormone from the pituitary.
5. ***Growth Hormone Release***: Endogenous growth hormone is released in physiologically relevant, pulsatile bursts. This hormone then enters systemic circulation and exerts its effects throughout the body.
6. ***IGF-1 Production***: In response to GH, the liver and other tissues increase the production of insulin-like growth factor 1 (IGF-1), which carries many of the growth hormone's anabolic and metabolic effects forward.
7. ***Target Tissue Effects***: GH and IGF-1 together stimulate lipolysis (breakdown of fat), especially targeting visceral adipose tissue. They also influence glucose metabolism, protein synthesis, and tissue regeneration.
8. ***Feedback Regulation***: The hypothalamic-pituitary axis then responds with feedback mechanisms to

regulate hormone levels, reducing the potential for unchecked production.

This sequence helps clarify why Tesamorelin's effects such as reductions in visceral fat develop progressively over weeks rather than days. The molecular chain of events relies on the body's orchestrated response, rather than overwhelming it with immediate, artificial hormone surges.

Signal Pathway Checklist for Identifying Direct and Indirect Physiological Effects

To systematically interrogate claims about what Tesamorelin might do, it's essential to distinguish between direct effects (those stemming from GHRH receptor activation and subsequent GH release) and indirect or secondary outcomes (effects resulting from downstream physiological changes).

A practical signal pathway checklist includes:

- Does the effect originate logically from increased endogenous growth hormone and IGF-1?
- Is the claimed physiological change supported by known properties of the GHRH-pituitary axis?
- Can the timeline of the effect (e.g., fat loss, improved metabolic markers) plausibly fit the gradual downstream impact typical of Tesamorelin's mode of action?

- Are feedback loops that normally suppress excess GH production intact, reducing the likelihood of runaway effects?
- Are there non-specific effects that might reflect more general metabolic shifts or influences of other hormone systems?

For example, a claim that Tesamorelin "rapidly increases muscle mass in days" doesn't align well with the established timeline of the hormonal cascade and likely signals exaggeration. In contrast, modest reductions in visceral fat over weeks of treatment are supported by the documented molecular pathway and observed in approval studies.

Table of Known Interactions with Other Hormones and Medication Classes

Tesamorelin, by virtue of its stimulation of the growth hormone axis, inevitably interacts with multiple hormonal pathways and may alter the effects of some medications. For the evidence-minded skeptic, grasping these connections is vital to parsing side effect profiles and potential drug interactions.

A summary table of relevant interactions is as follows:

Table 2: Table of Known Interactions with Other Hormones and Medication Classes

Hormone/ Medication Class	Nature of Interaction	Clinical Significance
Insulin & Oral Hypoglycemics	GH and IGF-1 can decrease insulin sensitivity	Potential for worsening glycemic control; monitor diabetics closely
Glucocorticoids	GH pathway can modulate cortisol action and vice versa	Doses of corticosteroids may need adjustment
Estrogens and Androgens	Sex steroids can influence IGF-1 and GH responsiveness	May impact baseline GH/IGF-1 levels
Pituitary Hormone Replacers	Overlapping mechanisms; changes in one may affect others	Complex feedback requires specialist oversight
Drugs affecting CYP enzymes	Minimal direct effect; Tesamorelin not primarily metabolized by CYP pathways	Reduced interaction compared to some other peptides
Antineoplastic Agents	GH axis stimulation may be contraindicated in malignancy contexts	Should NOT be co-administered in active cancers

The most clinically relevant interaction is with glucose-lowering medications. Tesamorelin-induced increases in GH often lead to reductions in insulin sensitivity, potentially unmasking glucose intolerance or precipitating new-onset diabetes especially in those already at risk.

This highlights the importance of baseline glucose monitoring and ongoing assessment during therapy. Other interactions, such as with sex steroids or glucocorticoids, are more nuanced, generally requiring oversight in those with complex endocrine backgrounds.

Model for Mapping the Boundaries of Current Mechanistic Understanding

Despite detailed knowledge of Tesamorelin's receptor-mediated action, there remain clear boundaries to what is mechanistically certain and what remains speculative. Recognizing these boundaries allows the skeptic to sort robust findings from preliminary or presumed effects.

Boundary mapping for Tesamorelin involves:

- ***Certainty at the Receptor Level***: There is strong, reproducible evidence for Tesamorelin's selectivity and agonism at GHRH receptors in the pituitary, resulting in reliable endogenous GH secretion in line with known physiological feedback.
- ***Reliability through the Hormonal Cascade***: The secondary production of IGF-1 mediated by GH's action on the liver is also well-established and supported by measurable effects in clinical use, such as reductions in visceral adipose tissue after regular administration.

- ***Well-documented Timeline***: The onset and magnitude of physiological effects—particularly fat reduction—align with the expected timescale for GH/IGF-1 mediated changes: moderate, progressive, and plateauing after several weeks of therapy.
- ***Defined Limits in Off-Target or Off-Label Mechanisms***: Data supporting Tesamorelin's roles outside of approved indications (e.g., general anti-aging, cognitive enhancement, rapid muscle-building) are less robust, and often based on extrapolated or preliminary findings. The mechanistic chain is much less clear outside the domain of fat reduction in HIV-associated lipodystrophy.
- ***Feedback and Risk Boundaries***: The body's natural feedback loops curtail excess hormone production, limiting some of the risks seen with exogenous GH therapies. However, situations that disturb these loops such as pituitary dysfunction, pre-existing hormone disorders, or malignancy may alter safety and efficacy, and reflect key boundaries of appropriate use.

Simply put, skepticism mandates confining strong claims about Tesamorelin to those effects supported by well-understood pathways. Approving authorities generally restrict claims and marketing to those outcomes such as visceral fat reduction in the target HIV population where the mechanistic evidence is matched by substantial clinical trial data.

Summary: Mapping for the Evidence-Seeker

For anyone evaluating the scientific basis of a Tesamorelin claim, this chapter provides a sequenced, evidence-based framework:

- Tesamorelin's effect is initiated at the GHRH receptor on the pituitary, with downstream induction of the growth hormone/IGF-1 axis.
- The molecular sequence from injection to target tissue effects is gradual and physiologically regulated, supporting only those outcomes compatible with known timescales and feedback systems.
- By laying out checkpoint questions and interaction tables, you can recognize when claims overstep mechanistic boundaries or rest on poorly substantiated speculation.
- Certain interactions, particularly with the glucose regulatory axis or in patients with underlying malignancy, introduce risk profiles that demand close monitoring or outright avoidance.
- The most reliable claims about Tesamorelin are those that fit both the mapped biological pathway and the tight constraints established by regulatory and clinical evidence.

Approaching Tesamorelin with a map of its mechanisms does more than satisfy scientific rigor. It empowers you to challenge unsupported assertions, ask smarter questions, and ensure that both risk and benefit remain tethered to what is genuinely known. This mechanistic lens is foundational for every subsequent step in this guide whether critiquing new studies, weighing clinical outcomes, or interrogating the inevitable marketing hype that surrounds this unique peptide.

Evidence Hierarchy for Tesamorelin Claims

Understanding the level and quality of evidence behind any claim about Tesamorelin is foundational for a well-reasoned, skeptical approach. Given the diversity of assertions in medical literature, professional marketing, and user anecdotes, it's crucial to distinguish between what is robustly supported, what is preliminary or suggestive, and what lacks credible substantiation altogether.

This chapter offers practical frameworks and tools to systematically classify Tesamorelin evidence, recognize biases, and avoid common pitfalls seen in the interpretation of peptide research.

Three-Tier Rating Framework for Preclinical, Clinical, and Postmarketing Evidence

The landscape of Tesamorelin data spans early laboratory findings to long-term human monitoring. To help you make sense of this spectrum, a three-tier hierarchy can be applied to nearly any claim:

Tier 1: Preclinical Evidence

This tier encompasses fundamental research performed in laboratory settings, cell cultures, animal studies, or in vitro assays. For Tesamorelin, preclinical data provided the first clues about its ability to mimic native growth hormone-releasing hormone (GHRH) and bind selectively to pituitary receptors.

However, results in non-human settings are always considered preliminary. While preclinical studies may demonstrate a plausible mechanism or reveal potential safety signals, they cannot reliably predict real-world effectiveness, optimal dosing, or human safety profiles.

Tier 2: Clinical Evidence

Clinical evidence represents the gold standard for evaluating therapies such as Tesamorelin. This encompasses randomized controlled trials (RCTs), cohort studies, and comparative group studies in human populations. For Tesamorelin, approval by regulatory authorities is grounded firmly in well-controlled clinical trials that demonstrated efficacy in reducing visceral adiposity in HIV-infected individuals with lipodystrophy.

These studies typically feature robust design, control arms, statistical analysis, and prespecified outcomes. The quality of clinical evidence varies, with RCTs providing the highest internal validity, followed by well-conducted observational studies.

Tier 3: Postmarketing Evidence

Once a product is released for prescription use, additional data accumulates via postmarketing surveillance, real-world evidence, and spontaneous reporting of benefits and adverse events. For Tesamorelin, this tier is crucial for identifying effects that might not emerge in smaller, tightly controlled studies. Postmarketing surveillance can reveal rare adverse effects, document off-label usage patterns, and evaluate long-term effectiveness and safety in broader patient populations. However, this evidence is often less controlled and more prone to confounders.

It is important to remember that claims based solely on preclinical or anecdotal postmarketing data should be viewed as hypothesis-generating, not definitive. A careful skeptic always weighs claims in light of the highest tier of available evidence.

Table Contrasting Study Types Relevant to Tesamorelin

Different types of research studies support claims about Tesamorelin, but not all are created equal. The following table contrasts commonly encountered study designs applied to Tesamorelin, their general strengths, and cautionary notes:

Table 3: Table Contrasting Study Types

Study Type	Typical Features	Strengths	Cautions/ Weaknesses
Randomized Controlled Trial (RCT)	Double-blind, placebo- or active-controlled, large sample size	Highest level for causality and bias minimization	Expensive, may exclude complex real-world populations; relatively short duration
Prospective Cohort Study	Follows groups assigned by exposure (Tesamorelin vs. none) through time	Captures real-world effectiveness and side effects over time	Prone to selection and confounding bias; less control vs. RCT
Case- Control Study	Retrospective, compares those with/without outcome	Efficient for rare adverse events	Sensitive to recall and selection bias; cannot establish causality
Case Report/ Series	Detailed account(s) of individual or small group outcomes	Useful for novel side effects or unique scenarios	No control group; cannot generalize, extremely limited validity
Postmarketing Surveillance	Aggregate data collected post-approval (registries, safety reporting)	Identifies long-term safety, infrequent risks	Passive data collection, underreporting, lack of denominator data

The bulk of Tesamorelin's approved claims such as visceral fat reduction in HIV-infected adults with lipodystrophy are based on multiple, well-powered RCTs, which set the bar for trustworthy evidence. In contrast, "real-world" use, anecdotal reports, or claims propagated in less formal settings often stem from case reports or uncontrolled observation, which are valuable starting points but do not warrant strong confidence.

Checklist for Recognizing Common Study Design Biases in Tesamorelin Literature

Even when a study proclaims exciting findings about Tesamorelin, the reliability of its conclusions can be threatened by multiple forms of bias. Applying a structured checklist can help identify these common traps:

- ☐ ***Is the Assignment Randomized?*** Non-random assignments open the door to selection bias, where groups differ in important confounding factors unrelated to Tesamorelin.
- ☐ Are the Study and Control Groups Well-Matched? Look for baseline similarity in age, underlying conditions, and other medications. Imbalances can distort apparent effects.
- ☐ Is Blinding Used? Investigator or participant awareness of allocation (Tesamorelin vs. placebo) can introduce expectation bias especially for subjective outcomes like self-reported well-being.

- ☐ ***Are Outcomes Clearly Defined and Measured Objectively?*** Objective endpoints (e.g., DEXA-measured changes in fat mass) are less prone to bias than subjective scales or “feelings” of improvement.
- ☐ ***What Proportion of Participants Completed the Study?*** High dropout rates threaten the validity of findings. Was intention-to-treat analysis performed, or were only those who completed the trial analyzed?
- ☐ ***Was There Pre-Registration and Transparency in Reporting?*** Studies registered before data collection and that report all prespecified endpoints provide greater confidence.
- ☐ ***Are Relevant Confounders Adjusted For?*** Known factors such as underlying metabolic conditions or co-administered drugs can skew results. Adjusted analyses are more trustworthy.
- ☐ ***Was the Participant Population Broad or Narrow?*** Narrowly selected populations may not reflect typical users, limiting generalizability.
- ☐ ***Are Results Statistically and Clinically Significant?*** A statistically significant change may be too small to matter in real life, scrutinize both the numbers and their practical impact.

Vigilantly applying these filters to both published studies and gray literature can prevent overreliance on sources that are built on methodological quicksand.

Template for Tracking Evidence Quality Supporting Each Claimed Effect

To systematically vet the many claims surrounding Tesamorelin, use a structured template to record core details for each purported benefit (or risk). Here's a practical sample table you can adapt:

Table 4: Template for Tracking Evidence

Claimed Effect	Tier of Evidence	Study Type (and N)	Control Used?	Objective Outcome	Risk of Bias?	Main Limitation(s)	Verdict on Credibility
Visceral fat reduction (HIV lipodystrophy)	Tier 2 (Clinical)	Multiple RCTs (n>800)	Placebo	DEXA scan	Low	Short duration	High
Reduced IGF-1 deficiency	Tier 2	RCTs, Cohort	Placebo	Serum IGF-1	Medium	Modest magnitude	Moderate
Improved insulin sensitivity	Tier 2/3	Observational, Postmarketing	None	HOMA-IR	High	Uncontrolled	Weak
Anti-aging benefit	Tier 1/3	Animal studies, case reports	None	Subjective	Very High	Anecdotal, low N	Not Supported

Filling out such a table forces clarity about the underlying nature of the supporting evidence, separating what is proven, plausible, or speculative regarding Tesamorelin's action.

Signal Detection Rules for Identifying Underpowered or Anecdotal Sources

With a flood of claims circulating online and in less rigorous formats, skeptics must develop "signal detection" habits to rapidly filter noise from valid evidence. These key rules tailored to Tesamorelin literature help identify warnings that a claim is built more on wishful thinking than substantiated performance:

1. ***Watch for Sample Size ("N")***: If a study or report presents findings from single individuals or only a handful of patients, treat conclusions as preliminary or purely hypothesis-generating.
2. ***Scrutinize Duration and Follow-Up***: Tesamorelin's physiological effects typically develop over weeks to months. Short-term claims or side effects appearing after a single dose should be interpreted with caution.
3. ***Look for Control Conditions***: Absence of a comparator group (placebo or standard therapy) leaves findings open to placebo effect and other confounders.
4. ***Assess for Selective or Cherry-Picked Reporting***: If only positive results are highlighted while negative or null outcomes are omitted, the risk of reporting bias is high.
5. ***Be Wary of Non-objective Outcomes***: Claims relying solely on subjective experiences, especially unblinded or uncontrolled, are vulnerable to significant bias.
6. ***Check for Replication***: A single, unpublished, or non-peer-reviewed study especially if outside the context of recognized indications should not be the basis for strong conclusions about Tesamorelin.

7. ***Follow the Journal and Investigator Lineage***: Research conducted in rigorous, peer-reviewed environments and by authors with transparency in funding or conflicts of interest carries more weight.
8. ***Consider Postmarketing Reports Cautiously***: Anecdotal side effect reports or claimed off-label benefits submitted voluntarily after market approval lack the methodological rigor of controlled studies and should be seen as signals requiring follow-up, not endpoints in themselves.

Practical Application: Navigating Real-World Claims About Tesamorelin

For everyday users, clinicians, or policy-makers encountering claims about Tesamorelin whether they are dramatic reports of rapid fat loss or dire warnings of unusual side effects, the tools and frameworks from this chapter allow swift, structured prioritization of credible evidence.

Suppose you read testimonials or blogs claiming Tesamorelin "produces rapid, visible fat loss within days." Applying your knowledge:

- Note that regulatory approval was based on RCTs showing meaningful change over several weeks, not days.

- Identify that reports of changes "within days" almost certainly derive from anecdotal or uncontrolled experience classified as anecdote, not evidence.
- Applying your evidence template, you flag this claim as Tier 3 (postmarketing anecdote), unsupported by robust trial or regulatory data.

If a publication discusses Tesamorelin's safety and reports rare adverse events, but the sample size is minimal or there is no comparator, use your detection checklist:

- Is the study size and design sufficient to detect truly rare risks?
- Were the adverse effects also observed in larger, controlled trials?
- Is the report hypothesis-generating or conclusive?

By insistently mapping every claim against these evidence hierarchies, design bias checklists, and detection rules, you empower yourself to separate reliable signals from marketing hype or wishful thinking. The end result: decisions and discussions around Tesamorelin grounded in the best available, carefully vetted scientific knowledge neither overly skeptical of robust evidence, nor unduly credulous toward questionable or premature reports.

This layered approach to evidence is not just academic rigor: it is a bulwark against being misled, ensuring that your evaluation of Tesamorelin always begins and ends with the question: "What is actually known, for whom, and with what degree of certainty?"

Efficacy Assessment Comparison Table

Evaluating Tesamorelin's clinical effectiveness is not simply a matter of believing the boldest claim or the largest anecdote. Instead, it requires a careful, structured approach to separate outcomes that are supported by rigorous FDA-approved evidence from those that float in the territory of off-label speculation.

This chapter supplies the practical tools and comparison frameworks to contextualize the promise and limitations of Tesamorelin, so any claim can be traced directly back to the solid ground of trial endpoints, regulatory standards, and the realities of medical versus experimental use.

Table of Clinical Outcomes: FDA-Approved Versus Unapproved Uses

The FDA's approval of Tesamorelin is narrowly defined, and this scope directly determines which claims are backed by robust clinical outcome data. When you see dramatic testimonials or hear about new "miracle" uses, it's crucial to quickly check which zone approved or unapproved a claim belongs to. Here is a concise side-by-side comparison table summarizing the primary endpoints established in well-controlled trials leading to approval, versus those proposed or promoted without such support:

Table 5: Table of Clinical Outcomes

Outcome/ Use	FDA-Approved for Tesamo-relin	Documen-ted in RCTs Supporting Approval	Investiga-tional or Unapproved Use	Supported by Controlled Evidence?
Reduction in visceral adipose tissue (VAT) in HIV-infected adults with lipodystrophy	Yes	Yes	No	Yes
General obesity or weight loss (non-HIV)	No	No	Sometimes proposed	No
Reduction in subcutaneous fat	No	Minor, not primary endpoint	Sometimes observed	Weak
Improved insulin sensitivity	No (possibly neutral/ negative)	Mixed; not a core primary endpoint	Frequently hypothesized	Mixed / Not established
Anti-aging benefits	No	Not a studied endpoint	Widely marketed off-label	No
Improved cardiovascu-lar risk markers	No	Not a core endpoint	Occasionally claimed	Unverified
Enhanced muscle growth	No	Not evaluated in approval studies	Promoted in some wellness circles	No

The clear, FDA-approved therapeutic role for Tesamorelin is the reduction of excess visceral fat in HIV-infected individuals suffering from lipodystrophy, as verified by consistent reductions in trunk and abdominal visceral fat on imaging studies during controlled clinical trials.

All other uses such as weight loss in the general population, anti-aging applications, or enhanced performance lack endorsement by either regulatory authorities or robust clinical trials. Claims of efficacy in these areas should be subject to high scrutiny and demand a stronger evidentiary burden.

List of Endpoint Measures in Tesamorelin Trials and Their Relevance

The clinical trials underpinning Tesamorelin's FDA approval are anchored to specific, objectively measurable endpoints. A clear understanding of these helps focus skepticism wherever a claim relies on vague or subjective benefits. The most common and relevant endpoint measures in key Tesamorelin studies are:

- ***Visceral Adipose Tissue (VAT) Volume***: Measured by CT or MRI imaging, VAT reduction is the gold-standard primary endpoint and the direct basis for regulatory approval for HIV-associated lipodystrophy. Reduction in VAT is associated with improved metabolic risk, but it is the change in this specific fat compartment, not general weight or subcutaneous fat, that is the target of Tesamorelin therapy.

- ***Subcutaneous Adipose Tissue (SAT) Volume***: Also measured by imaging, but while sometimes reduced, this is not the main study endpoint and not the basis for approval or clinical decision-making for Tesamorelin.
- ***Waist Circumference***: Used as a practical proxy for VAT reduction, but less precise than imaging. It is often reported as a secondary endpoint.
- ***Serum IGF-1 (Insulin-Like Growth Factor 1)***: Tesamorelin induces the release of growth hormone, which in turn increases IGF-1. Normalization of IGF-1 levels may be used to confirm biochemical efficacy, but clinical benefit is attributed to changes in VAT rather than IGF-1 alone.
- ***Glucose and Insulin Homeostasis (Ex: HOMA-IR)***: These are metabolic indicators collected in some studies to monitor potential impacts on insulin resistance. A key safety concern, as altered glucose handling is a known risk with any growth hormone–modulating therapy.
- ***Lipid Profiles (Cholesterol, Triglycerides)***: Examined as secondary endpoints to assess any benefit (or risk) to cardiovascular biomarkers, though findings are generally less consistent and not central to FDA approval.

- ***Adverse Event Incidence***: While not an "efficacy" endpoint, reporting of side effect profiles is included in all pivotal studies and vital to a full risk-benefit assessment.

Understanding these endpoints allows you to immediately spot when a claimed benefit (like "increased muscle mass" or "significant weight loss in healthy subjects") was never objectively measured in high-quality Tesamorelin trials, and therefore is not FDA-validated nor supported by the primary literature base.

Criteria for Interpreting Statistically and Clinically Meaningful Changes

It is not enough to simply see numbers move in the right direction. Any skeptic must distinguish between effects that are statistically significant unlikely to be due to chance and those that are clinically meaningful large enough to actually matter to a patient or practitioner.

Some key criteria for Tesamorelin efficacy include:

- ***Magnitude of Change***: For VAT, clinical trials generally expect a reduction of at least 8% to 20% to be considered meaningful for individual patient health. Statistically smaller reductions, even if they reach $p<0.05$, may have little practical benefit.

- ***Duration of Benefit***: Temporary changes that disappear after a few weeks are less meaningful than those maintained with ongoing use, and especially if demonstrated after stopping therapy (sustainability).
- ***Baseline to Endpoint Shift***: Look for mean or median delta values in primary endpoints (i.e., average VAT reduced), not just percentage of "responders." Group averages should show clear, clinically relevant movement.
- ***Comparator and Control***: True effect size should be judged against a placebo or active control not just baseline—since placebo may produce considerable perceived change.
- ***Safety-Tolerability Balance***: Any benefit, however statistically robust, should be weighed against incident rate and severity of side effects (e.g., impaired glucose tolerance, local injection reactions), which can diminish the net value of the result.
- ***Patient-Reported Quality of Life***: Only count subjective improvements if collected using validated, blinded measures as secondary endpoints.

When assessing Tesamorelin claims, always check for direct reporting of these criteria in clinical trial results. For instance, a 15% absolute VAT reduction sustained over 26 weeks and significantly greater than placebo, with an acceptable side effect profile, is both a statistically and clinically meaningful outcome. Conversely, a "trend" toward improved well-being without objective or replicated measurement carries little weight.

Template for Comparing Efficacy in Subgroups

The value of Tesamorelin may differ between populations, a critical factor often disregarded in casual or non-clinical claims. Here is a clear template to compare documented efficacy in approved subgroups (e.g., HIV-associated lipodystrophy) with unstudied or off-label contexts (e.g., general, non-HIV obesity):

Table 6: Template for Comparing Efficacy in Subgroups

Subgroup/ Context	Evidence Type	Measured Efficacy (Primary Endpoint)	Clinical Relevance	FDA Status	Notes
HIV+ with lipodystrophy	Multiple RCTs, FDA review	VAT reduction: 8-20% (mean); increased IGF-1; improvement seen in 12–26 weeks	High: meets regulatory and guideline thresholds	Approved	Largest evidence base
Non-HIV general obesity	Limited, uncontrolled data	Not reliably measured; effect size unknown	Unknown/ Likely minimal	Not approved	Claims unsupported
Individuals seeking "anti-aging" or muscle gain	Anecdotal, case reports	None or subjective; endpoints not assessed	No proven effect; safety unclear	Not approved	Off-label marketing only

This table framework allows any consumer or decision-maker to explicitly trace which subgroup is truly supported by data, rapidly flagging when enthusiasm outstrips evidence. For example, in the HIV+ lipodystrophy group, sustained VAT reduction is robustly documented in multiple trials, while for "anti-aging" or "fat burning" in healthy adults, genuine efficacy evidence is absent or purely anecdotal.

Checklist for Weighing Duration, Sustainability, and Size of Effects

When making practical decisions about Tesamorelin claims, a simple checklist helps ensure you don't overlook core questions about the real-world value of a documented effect:

- ☐ Was the endpoint measured over a sufficiently long period (e.g., 12–26 weeks)?
- ☐ Did the effect persist through the entire treatment duration, or was it lost after cessation?
- ☐ What was the absolute versus relative magnitude of the benefit e.g., how many centimeters from baseline, rather than just percent change?
- ☐ Are reported outcomes adjusted for control/placebo, or are they uncontrolled trends?
- ☐ How do dropout rates or adverse event–related discontinuations impact the results and generalizability?
- ☐ Are there published follow-up data showing durability of benefit after discontinuation, or do effects quickly regress?
- ☐ For multi-point endpoints (fat volume, IGF-1 increase, glucose parameters), are improvements consistent

across all measures, or isolated to a single, potentially less-relevant one?

- ☐ Is the effect size large enough to shift risk categories (e.g., moving a patient from "high" to "medium" VAT risk) or merely reflect a small, non-transformative numeric reduction?
- ☐ Do subgroup analyses suggest greater benefit for certain ages, sexes, or clinical backgrounds, or are effects uniform only in narrowly selected trial populations?

For Tesamorelin, the best evidence shows that VAT reduction occurs gradually over several months and is sustained only with continued therapy cessation leads to a gradual return toward baseline values. Immediate, dramatic, or permanent effects are not substantiated in any RCT, and all robust claims must reflect this reality.

Putting the Table to Work: How to Use This Matrix for Any New Tesamorelin Claim

Whenever you encounter a new assertion about Tesamorelin whether in a medical paper, a promotional ad, or peer discussion consult this set of tables and checklists. Demand to see:

- The exact endpoint(s) measured
- The subgroup under study and how it compares to the population described

- The duration and sustainability of benefit
- The size (absolute and relative) of documented changes
- All caveats regarding site effects, study design, and withdrawal rates

This commitment to granular, transparent, criteria-driven evaluation is your strongest defense against being swayed by incomplete, exaggerated, or flatly unsupported Tesamorelin efficacy claims. The more you practice these objective habits, the easier it becomes to map real clinical meaning onto the crowded, often noisy space of peptide therapy marketing.

When you root your assessment in what has actually been documented through FDA-standard trials, pre-specified endpoints, and meaningful durations you maintain both fairness and rigor, never losing sight of the true measure of Tesamorelin's genuine clinical value.

Safety, Risks, and Adverse Effects Framework

A skeptical and systematic approach to Tesamorelin must place safety concerns front and center. No claim about benefit carries real weight unless you can simultaneously understand and monitor potential risks, side effects, and gaps in knowledge that may influence your risk–benefit calculation.

This chapter provides you with a clear, data-driven framework for charting the true side effect landscape, recognizing red flags for severe reactions or misuse, benchmarking trial data against real-world outcomes, and tracking emerging safety issues as the evidence base develops over time.

Table of Documented Side Effects by Frequency and Severity (Short and Long Term)

Understanding Tesamorelin's adverse effect profile requires separating the quantifiable from the anecdotal, the mild and common from the rare yet serious. Proper skepticism starts with a structured overview of what has been consistently reported in clinical research, FDA submissions, and post-approval safety monitoring.

Side effects of Tesamorelin can be broken down by frequency (common, less common, rare) and by severity (mild, moderate, severe). This helps calibrate both expectations for typical users and vigilance for emerging harms.

Common side effects (short-term, usually not severe):

- ***Injection site reactions***: Including redness, itching, pain, swelling, or rash at the injection area. These are among the most frequent adverse events observed in both clinical trials and real-world prescribing. Most are mild and resolve without intervention.
- ***Muscle pain or discomfort***: Mild myalgias can occur, often transient and self-limited.
- ***Joint pain (arthralgia)***: Episodic, and in most cases, not disabling or persistent.
- ***Headache***: Mild to moderate intensity, generally not requiring discontinuation.
- ***Peripheral edema (swelling, especially in the lower limbs)***: This is not uncommon with growth hormone–modulating treatments and should be monitored, particularly in users with cardiovascular risk factors.

Less common or more clinically notable side effects:

- ***Hypersensitivity/allergic reactions***: Including urticaria (hives), angioedema, and in rare cases, anaphylaxis. Any sign of acute swelling, respiratory difficulty, or generalized rash demands immediate attention.
- ***Glucose intolerance/altered glycemic control***: Growth hormone analogs can disrupt insulin sensitivity, potentially unmasking or worsening diabetes. Blood glucose monitoring is especially important for those with prediabetes or established diabetes.
- ***Injection site lipoatrophy or lipodystrophy***: Fat loss or redistribution at frequent injection sites, though rare, may appear over longer-term use.
- ***Fluid retention/severe edema***: Cases of more pronounced fluid retention may evolve, particularly in those at cardiovascular risk.

Rare but severe or long-term risks:

- ***Neoplasia/Unmasked Malignancy***: While direct causation has not been firmly established, theoretical concerns exist for accelerated growth of latent tumors, particularly in patients with undiagnosed malignancy. Long-term human safety data are still accruing, and any sign of unexplained new symptoms warrants careful evaluation.
- ***Pituitary or hypothalamic dysfunction***: By design, Tesamorelin stimulates pituitary growth hormone release, and there is a theoretical risk of functional

disruption in the hormonal axis, though documented cases are extremely rare.

- ***Acute hypersensitivity (anaphylaxis)***: Though exceedingly uncommon, labeling still mandates vigilance for rapid worsening allergic reactions.

Here is a summary table synthesizing frequency and severity:

Table 7: Summary Table Synthesizing Frequency and Severity

Adverse Effect	Frequency	Severity (Typical)	Short- or Long-Term	Notes
Injection site reactions	Common	Mild	Short-term	Most cases self-limited
Muscle/ joint pain	Common	Mild–Moderate	Short-term	Rarely interferes with use
Headache	Common	Mild–Moderate	Short-term	
Peripheral edema	Common	Mild–Moderate	Short-term	Monitor if cardiac risk present
Glucose intolerance	Less common	Moderate–Severe	Short/ Long-term	Monitor in diabetes/ prediabetes
Hypersensi-tivity (mild)	Uncommon	Moderate	Short-term	Can appear as rash or hives
Severe allergic reaction	Rare	Severe	Short-term	Immediate medical attention required
Lipoatrophy/ lipodystro-phy	Rare	Mild–Moderate	Long-term	Associated with repeated injection
Tumor growth/ unmasking	Very rare/ theoretical	Severe	Long-term	Remains a theoretical concern

Always review updated safety labeling and clinical documentation, as this table is built from both pivotal trial and post-marketing surveillance data.

Comparison between clinical trial safety outcomes and real-world postmarketing data

Clinical trials provide the initial, controlled assessment of Tesamorelin's safety usually in carefully screened populations and under close monitoring. Postmarketing (real-world) data, however, expands this view, often revealing rare or longer-term side effects not captured in trials.

Clinical trial findings typically report:

- High rates of mild to moderate injection site reactions, confirming that local tolerability issues are nearly ubiquitous but rarely prompt discontinuation.
- Modest increases in muscle/joint pain, headache, and edema, with very low discontinuation rates for these symptoms.
- Increases in blood glucose and new-onset diabetes infrequently, but with enough incidence to merit regular glucose monitoring, especially in at-risk groups.

Postmarketing experience highlights several trends:

- While severe allergic reactions remain uncommon, real-world settings report these events outside the controlled context of trials, potentially under less vigilant monitoring.
- Occasional reports of injection site lipoatrophy, more often in users who do not rotate injection sites properly, a detail less likely to appear in closely supervised clinical studies.
- Glucose homeostasis issues, in some cases leading to more significant metabolic complications than observed in the relatively healthy trial cohorts.
- No large safety signals for tumor growth or new neoplasms, but continued monitoring is necessary, as approval-period trial durations did not capture very long-term use.

Key comparison takeaway: For most users in either context, Tesamorelin's side effect burden remains predominantly mild and predictable, but clinicians and consumers must be vigilant for rare but significant risks. Greater frequency of metabolic effects in real-world reports suggests a need for ongoing glycemic monitoring and individualized risk assessment.

Checklist for Red Flags Indicating Misuse or Adverse Event Escalation

While most Tesamorelin users will experience only mild, manageable side effects, certain warning signs suggest either misuse or the escalation toward serious adverse reactions. Early identification allows for prompt intervention.

Use this red flag checklist:

- ☐ Rapid, widespread swelling, difficulty breathing, or generalized hives after injection—potential sign of anaphylaxis, always a medical emergency.
- ☐ Marked, persistent elevation in blood glucose or new symptoms of hyperglycemia (increased thirst, urination, fatigue), especially in those without prior diabetes these merit re-evaluation of the risk–benefit calculus.
- ☐ Sustained or severe pain, induration, or changes (dimpling/fat loss) at injection sites may represent local complications or early lipoatrophy.
- ☐ Unexplained headaches or vision changes rarely, intracranial hypertension may develop, and persistent symptoms require prompt assessment.
- ☐ Appearance of new lumps, masses, or unexplained symptoms is a possible (though rare) indicator of unmasking a pre-existing neoplasm.
- ☐ Use of non-standard doses or administration methods ("stacking," frequent off-label escalations) greatly increases risk for unstudied side effects or toxicities.
- ☐ Ignoring or self-medicating through persistent or worsening adverse effects rather than pausing or seeking medical review.

If any of these red flags appear, Tesamorelin should be held, and proper evaluation sought before resuming therapy.

Rules for Distinguishing Likely Versus Speculative Risks Based on Strength of Evidence

In analyzing safety claims about Tesamorelin, it is vital to separate what is well-documented from what is anecdotal or entirely theoretical. A rational, skeptical approach assigns greater weight to risks consistently reported in structured studies and sanctioned by regulatory agencies, and less to concerns that lack empirical backing or arise solely from mechanistic speculation.

Rules for evidence-based risk assessment with Tesamorelin:

- ***Likely (well-documented) risks*** are those repeatedly reported in phase 3 trials, labeled by regulatory authorities, and observed in real-world surveillance: e.g., injection site reactions, mild peripheral edema, occasional glucose intolerance.
- Probable but less common risks are recognized by labeling but rare in trials such as lipoatrophy with improper injection technique, or severe allergic reactions where mechanistic plausibility and real-world cases both exist.

- ***Speculative or theoretical risks*** (e.g., tumor acceleration in the absence of existing neoplasia, long-term pituitary dysfunction in a healthy adult) should not be dismissed, but must be recognized as extrapolations without confirmation by hard outcome data.
- ***Anecdotal or unsubstantiated risks*** (arising from secondhand reports, one-off patient claims, or extreme interpretations of animal data) should be given little weight until substantiated in larger series or at least consistent case reports.
- ***Magnitude and quality of evidence***: Place greatest trust in safety signals confirmed by multiple, well-designed human studies and large postmarketing cohorts. Claims based solely on isolated events, mechanistic concern, or preclinical models need continued tracking but not immediate alarm.

Practical application: If new side effects or risks for Tesamorelin are promoted but do not appear in regulatory labeling, major trial data, or systematic postmarket surveillance, regard them as unproven pending further data.

Protocol for Tracking Unresolved Safety Questions and Monitoring Updates

The science around Tesamorelin, especially long-term risks and very rare events remains open to revision as more people use the medication and more data are collected. To maintain a genuinely evidence-driven, skepticism-based perspective, adopt a living protocol for tracking open safety questions and remaining abreast of updates.

A stepwise protocol:

1. ***Maintain a running list of unresolved safety questions***: For example, "Does long-term Tesamorelin increase any cancer risk in healthy adults?" or "What are the effects of chronic metabolic changes on cardiovascular endpoints?"
2. ***Check formal safety update sources regularly***: For example, search FDA or Health Canada safety bulletins, drug labels, and peer-reviewed pharmacovigilance studies every 6–12 months.
3. ***Review summaries from large registries or postmarketing surveillance reports***: These can reveal rare or late-emerging safety signals not seen in initial trials.
4. ***Track trial registry databases (e.g., clinicaltrials.gov) for new, ongoing, or completed Tesamorelin safety studies***: Especially those extending follow-up periods or expanding to new populations.
5. ***Log relevant adverse event reports from peer-reviewed journals***: Record both the claimed effect and the context (dose, duration, population).

6. ***Regularly revisit and update your table of documented side effects***: Compare new data against prior consensus, and explicitly mark where uncertainty has narrowed or increased.

By adhering to this protocol, the skeptic ensures that Tesamorelin safety assessments are always grounded in the most current, direct, and robust evidence possible. Unresolved questions should never be dismissed by default; they should remain "open liabilities" rather than points of certainty.

The landscape of Tesamorelin safety is neither static nor free from ambiguity. The best safeguard against overconfidence, marketing manipulation, or inappropriate use is a habit of systematic risk evaluation integrating controlled trial data, postmarketing surveillance, red flag vigilance, a clear hierarchy for evidence weight, and a living protocol for ongoing monitoring.

By insisting that all safety claims or concerns about Tesamorelin meet these standards, you protect yourself from both alarmist speculation and dangerous complacency. This is the disciplined, responsible pathway to informed, practical decision-making in the real-world context of Tesamorelin therapy.

Trade-off Analysis and Decision Criteria

Evaluating whether Tesamorelin is appropriate in a particular context involves more than just tallying benefits against risks. A disciplined, skepticism-based process asks: Are the trade-offs acceptable in this scenario, for this individual, with these goals? This chapter delivers the tools you need to move from vague impressions to a repeatable, explicit analysis so your decisions about Tesamorelin are systematic, rational, and resilient to hype or misplaced optimism.

Framework for Weighing Benefit vs Risk in Common Use Scenarios

To perform a meaningful trade-off analysis with Tesamorelin, start by explicitly outlining both its supported benefits and its documented risks for the specific clinical scenario in question. Tesamorelin is most commonly used and approved for the treatment of HIV-associated lipodystrophy, where it has demonstrated measurable reduction in abdominal (visceral) fat in affected patients. The benefit, in this setting, is not simply cosmetic but includes improvement of a risk factor associated with metabolic and cardiovascular complications.

Yet every benefit comes with trade-offs. For Tesamorelin, side effects from mild injection site reactions to metabolic disturbances and rare hypersensitivity must be considered not in the abstract, but in relation to the context and magnitude of benefit projected for the patient.

Key elements of a rational benefit–risk framework for Tesamorelin in common scenarios:

1. Define the clinical or wellness outcome you aim to affect (e.g., reduction in visceral fat, improvement in metabolic risk).
2. Identify the magnitude and certainty of benefit (what percent of patients experience target outcomes, and how large are these effects?).
3. Quantify the likelihood and severity of side effects or complications (both common and rare) based on the best available data.
4. Consider the duration of use and time to onset of benefit since some improvements may take weeks to manifest, while certain risks can appear early or with prolonged treatment.
5. Map out alternatives (including non-pharmacologic and pharmacologic) addressing the same goal.

With this information at hand, a meaningful, individualized benefit–risk balance begins to emerge.

Decision Criteria Table for Identifying When Trade-offs May Exceed Typical Thresholds

To distill complex trade-offs into practical decisions, use a criteria table that flags when the trade-off balance tips against Tesamorelin use for a given patient or context. The following decision criteria table specific to Tesamorelin's evidence base helps clarify when to proceed, pause, or seek alternatives:

Table 8: Decision Criteria Table

Criterion	Proceed with Tesamorelin	Pause or Reconsider	Consider Alternatives
Indication	Clear, approved (e.g., HIV lipodystrophy)	Off-label, weak evidence for benefit	Non-supported or experimental use
Patient Risk Profile	Low-moderate, comorbidities manageable	Significant metabolic, cardiac, or allergic risks	Very high or uncontrolled comorbidities
Severity of Baseline Condition	High impact on health/QOL	Mild or cosmetic concerns only	No clear burden from target condition
Previous Response to Similar Agents	No issues with GH analogs	Prior severe adverse effects	History of critical complications
Likelihood of Benefit	High, based on clinical data	Modest/ uncertain, mixed evidence	Minimal or anecdotal only
Side Effect Profile	Mild, predictable,	Early severe reactions or	High frequency of severe

	manageable	loss of tolerability	reactions
Ability to Monitor & Follow Up	Reliable monitoring possible	Limited monitoring, adherence concerns	No feasible ongoing safety/effect monitoring

If two or more criteria fall in the "Pause" or "Consider Alternatives" columns, the trade-offs with Tesamorelin may exceed the typical threshold for prudent use. This table is meant to be revisited at every critical juncture or if new information arises (e.g., unexpected side effects, updated clinical guidelines).

Checklist of Patient Factors That Influence Risk–Benefit Calculations for Tesamorelin

Because Tesamorelin's effects and side effect profile are influenced by individual factors, it is prudent to systematize a checklist for personalizing the trade-off analysis:

- ☐ Medical history of diabetes, prediabetes, or insulin resistance (heightens risk for glucose dysregulation)
- ☐ Cardiovascular disease or risk factors (warrants increased monitoring of edema and metabolic effects)
- ☐ Personal or family history of cancer/neoplasms (theoretical concern for growth hormone–dependent tumor stimulation)
- ☐ History of allergic reactions or hypersensitivity events, especially to peptide drugs (raises risk for adverse events)

- ☐ State of hepatic and renal function (potential effects on drug metabolism and clearance)
- ☐ Current medications or therapies (potential for drug–drug interactions, especially those affecting the pituitary or metabolic axis)
- ☐ Age and physiological reserve older individuals and the frail may have altered response or reduced side effect tolerance
- ☐ Ability and willingness to comply with injection protocol and ongoing monitoring requirements
- ☐ Previous experiences or outcomes with growth hormone–releasing analogs
- ☐ Likelihood or intention regarding off-label or supratherapeutic use, which may skew anticipated risk–benefit ratios

Each factor modifies the baseline trade-off. For example, a patient with unstable diabetes requires far more intensive glucose surveillance and may find risk outweighing benefit, while an individual without metabolic risk but with severe HIV-associated lipodystrophy may stand to gain more with manageable downside.

Flowchart for Integrating Goals, Alternatives, and Non-Pharmacy Strategies

A trade-off analysis blunted by tunnel vision, that is, only considering Tesamorelin often overlooks effective, lower-risk pathways to the same goal. A robust approach integrates alternative options, escalating only when necessary.

Here is a step-by-step flowchart for navigating Tesamorelin versus alternatives:

1. Start by clearly defining the primary outcome goal (e.g., reduction of visceral fat, improved metabolic profile).
2. List all appropriate, evidence-based interventions:
    - Non-pharmacy strategies (dietary change, exercise, behavioral modification targeting fat reduction)
    - Other pharmacologic options (standard GH analogs, if indicated, or alternative treatments targeted to root cause)
    - Tesamorelin, if specifically indicated

1. Assess for contraindications or non-candidates for each method (e.g., inability to exercise, intolerance to other medication classes).
2. Evaluate likelihood and timeline of benefit for each option (Tesamorelin typically requires weeks for measurable effect).
3. Consider the risk and burden of each option (side effect profile, monitoring, cost, inconvenience).
4. Rank options based on net expected benefit (benefit minus risk and burden).

5. Make selection and outline a monitoring plan, including decision points for switching or discontinuing the chosen intervention if predefined thresholds are crossed (e.g., unacceptable side effects, insufficient benefit after trial period).

This process keeps the focus broad and patient-centered, ensuring that Tesamorelin is considered within a comprehensive solution set.

Template for Gathering Baseline Data to Inform Ongoing Re-evaluation

A central tenet of skepticism-based medicine is ongoing, data-driven re-evaluation rather than "set-and-forget." Before and during Tesamorelin use, systematic data collection enables informed mid-course corrections—or discontinuation if the trade-offs worsen.

Use this structured template for baseline and ongoing re-evaluation:

Baseline Data Points:

- Target symptom(s) and/or measurable health outcome(s) (e.g., baseline visceral fat measure)
- Weight, BMI, waist circumference
- Fasting blood glucose and hemoglobin A1c
- Lipid profile (cholesterol, triglycerides)
- Blood pressure

- History of allergic reactions, especially to medications or injectables
- Current medications and supplements
- History of cancer or endocrine disorders
- Patient's goals and acceptability of possible risk levels
- Frequency and severity of pre-existing musculoskeletal symptoms (to differentiate from new-onset side effects)
- Ability and readiness to adhere to monitoring schedule and injection regimen

Ongoing Data Points (to be collected at regular intervals, e.g., every 1–3 months):

- Changes in target symptom(s) or outcome measure(s)
- Incidence and severity of side effects (documented with date and context)
- Blood glucose trends and any development of new glycemic abnormalities
- Injection site assessment
- New health conditions or notable changes in existing diagnoses
- Patient-reported tolerability and satisfaction
- Assessment of continued appropriateness based on new guidelines or evolving clinical evidence

These data elements provide the anchor for "go/no-go" decisions at each follow-up. Systematic documentation prevents emotion or anecdotal memory from crowding out rigorous assessment.

Practical Application and Summary

Making a decision about Tesamorelin demands more than accepting an expert's word or chasing a promising testimonial. Instead, it involves enacting a repeatable system—defining goals, understanding the evidence, explicitly weighing pros and cons, referencing clear thresholds for acceptability, and re-checking both data and assumptions along the way.

<u>Key steps in a skeptic's trade-off analysis:</u>

- Frame the intended benefit of Tesamorelin in the specific context (e.g., treating HIV-associated lipodystrophy, not generic "fat loss").
- Consult trial and postmarketing evidence to assess both chance and size of benefit and the risks most relevant to the individual at hand.
- Utilize a structured criteria table to clarify when trade-offs cease to make sense for a given patient.
- Incorporate a thorough checklist of patient-specific factors to personalize risk–benefit.
- Consider all reasonable alternatives, including those that do not involve medication.
- Collect robust baseline and ongoing data to ensure that theoretical benefit translates to real-world experience,

and to enable course correction or cessation if side effects, poor efficacy, or new risks emerge.

The skeptical approach does not mean rejecting Tesamorelin out of hand; instead, it means granting it a fair, evidence-weighted trial, embedded in ongoing evaluation, and always subject to revision as new evidence or outcomes arise. In this way, users and clinicians can move beyond guesswork to make judicious and defensible choices, grounded in both data and lived response, throughout every stage of Tesamorelin consideration and use.

Marketing, Hype, and Myth-Busting Ruleset

Tesamorelin occupies an unusual position in the medical and wellness marketplace: it is a specialized prescription peptide with well-documented benefits for specific clinical populations, yet it is often promoted with bold marketing, ambiguous promises, and persistent myths.

Understanding how to sift truth from hype is an essential skill for anyone considering or discussing Tesamorelin. This chapter equips you with practical tools to dissect claims, recognize misleading patterns, and independently verify the foundations of what you read or hear about Tesamorelin.

List of Common Marketing Claims and How to Flag Unsupported Language

When encountering information about Tesamorelin, especially outside reputable clinical settings, you'll likely notice certain patterns in marketing promises. Here are some of the most common types of claims and language features to scrutinize for lack of adequate support:

1. ***"Rapid Body Transformation"***: Phrases claiming visible or dramatic body changes in weeks without specific details about the population, measurement method, or timescale are red flags. While some patients may experience reductions in visceral adiposity, this typically occurs over months and is supported mainly in the context of HIV-associated lipodystrophy, not for general weight loss or fitness enhancement.
2. ***"Guaranteed Fat Loss"***: Any assertion that Tesamorelin works in all users, or that results are guaranteed regardless of underlying condition, is not reflective of the actual clinical evidence. Benefits are notably demonstrated in select populations, with varying individual responses.
3. ***"Anti-Aging Peptide"***: Claims that Tesamorelin slows aging, boosts youthfulness, or broadly reverses hormonal aging are unsubstantiated by robust human trials. While Tesamorelin increases growth hormone levels, approved uses remain highly targeted.
4. ***"Safe for Everyone, No Side Effects"***: Language that minimizes side effects or suggests broad safety is misleading. Tesamorelin has well-documented risks, including injection site reactions, edema, glucose abnormalities, and other side effects.
5. ***"Research-Proven for Muscle Growth"***: Statements presenting Tesamorelin as a muscle-building drug for

athletes or bodybuilders frequently overstate the available evidence. Its principal role, as demonstrated in research, is the reduction of visceral fat rather than direct anabolic effects in healthy subjects.

How to Flag Unsupported Language:

- Look for vague qualifiers like "may," "could," "proven," or "revolutionary" without direct references to clinical studies.
- Demand context: Which population? What timeframe? What clinical endpoints?
- Question absolutes: If a claim uses "always," "guaranteed," or "risk-free," additional skepticism is warranted.
- Check for citations: Are specific peer-reviewed studies or regulatory approvals referenced, and do these truly support the claim?

Table of Popular Myths Versus Evidence-Based Conclusions

Sorting myth from fact is crucial for sound clinical and personal decision-making. The table below contrasts some of the most widespread beliefs with evidence-supported conclusions about Tesamorelin:

Table 9: Popular Myths Versus Evidence-Based Conclusions

Popular Myth	Evidence-Based Conclusion
Tesamorelin works equally well for everyone	Benefits are best documented in HIV-associated lipodystrophy, with varying results in other populations and limited high-quality evidence for general weight loss.
No side effects or safety concerns	Documented side effects include edema, glucose intolerance, injection site reactions, and more; safety requires close monitoring.
Results are instantaneous	Clinically significant fat reduction usually requires 12–26 weeks; changes are gradual, not immediate.
Tesamorelin can be used as an anti-aging therapy	No robust clinical trial data supports its use as an anti-aging agent; off-label claims lack high-quality evidence.
It's approved for general obesity or bodybuilding	Regulatory approvals are specific to HIV lipodystrophy; general obesity and performance claims go beyond official indications.

Rules for Decoding Indirect, Exaggerated, or Ambiguous Benefit Statements

Tesamorelin marketing often employs language that is technically true on a narrow point but misleading in overall implication. Here's a codified method to see through such statements:

1. **Identify the Specific Benefit**

   Pinpoint what is actually being claimed. Is it reduction in visceral fat, improved metabolic health, or something broader and less defined?

2. **Find the Measured Endpoint and Population**

   Ask: Has this benefit been measured in controlled settings? Was it observed in HIV patients, in healthy volunteers, or another group?

3. **Note the Timeline and Magnitude**

   Ambiguous promises often ignore how long it takes to see results, their size, or their durability. Ask for specifics: How many weeks? What degree of change?

4. **Distinguish Clinical Significance From Statistical Changes**

   Not all reported differences are meaningful for actual health outcomes.

5. **Watch for "Science Washing"**

   Marketing may refer to "studies show" or "clinically tested" without naming the study or spelling out whether the same magnitude/effect applies to the marketed scenario. Cross-check whether cited studies actually support the scope and context of the claim.

6. **Spot Overgeneralization**

   Claims like "Tesamorelin improves body composition" are often true only within specific, well-defined populations and for certain measures. Generalizing beyond HIV lipodystrophy, for example, stretches the evidence base.

Checklist of Sources That Frequently Perpetuate Misinformation About Tesamorelin

Certain types of outlets or communicators consistently spread unsupported or exaggerated statements regarding Tesamorelin. Here is a checklist of sources that demand extra caution:

- ***Supplement and "Wellness" Retail Sites***: These often market Tesamorelin directly to consumers, ignoring prescription-only status and touting universal benefits, while minimizing mention of risks.
- ***Social Media Influencers***: Influencers in the realms of fitness, bodybuilding, or anti-aging sometimes exaggerate Tesamorelin's relevance to general health, youth, or attractiveness for likes and affiliate sales.
- ***Unregulated Online Pharmacies***: Sites selling Tesamorelin without prescriptions may present it as a safe, simple solution for weight management or muscle gain, often omitting warnings and regulatory details.
- ***Commercial Health Blogs***: Articles lacking author credentials, primary references, or clear

conflict-of-interest disclosures often restate others' marketing without critical analysis.

- ***Anonymous Forums and Testimonials***: Personal accounts or anecdotal "success stories" can amplify isolated experiences and ignore the importance of representative, systematic study data.
- ***Vague Science News Summaries***: Press releases or diluted summaries may imply that advances in Tesamorelin's understanding or approval cover many uses, when approvals are actually very restricted.

Protocol for Tracing the Origin of a Claim Through Marketing and Scientific Literature

Learning to verify the root of any assertion about Tesamorelin protects you against the spread of misinformation and helps ensure decisions are evidence-based. Here's a step-by-step protocol for claim tracing:

1. ***Record the Exact Claim***: Write down the full statement, noting the source type (ad, article, influencer, etc.) and what outcome or effect is being implied.
2. ***Check for Citations or References***: Is a primary research study, clinical guideline, or regulatory announcement cited? If not, be highly cautious.
3. ***Locate the Primary Study or Authority***: Use citation details to find the actual research prefer studies

catalogued on PubMed, major medical journals, or health regulatory websites.

4. ***Ensure the Study's Population, Design, and Results Match the Claim***: Investigate whether the outcomes in the primary study reflect the marketed claim: for example, was Tesamorelin studied in healthy volunteers or only in HIV-positive populations? What results were actually measured—fat loss, well-being, safety? Over what duration?
5. ***Check Approval Status***: Verify whether the use claimed has been approved by health authorities for that indication, or if it is experimental or off-label.
6. ***Identify Any Extrapolation or Omission***: Assess whether the claim omits side effects, timeframes, special monitoring needs, or caveats. Mark any disconnect between the claim scope and the study specifics.
7. ***Document any Gaps or Overextensions***: Note when a chain ends in a press release, animal study, or short-term surrogate endpoint instead of a robust trial. Mark the claim as insufficiently backed if it fails the test of direct, high-quality evidence for the stated benefit and population.
8. ***Compare Across Multiple Authoritative Sources***: Look for consensus (or lack thereof) from regulatory sites, published reviews, and established clinical

guidelines to ensure findings are not isolated or prematurely reported.

Applying this protocol ensures that each step in the logical path from marketing or hearsay to scientific substantiation is visible, accountable, and analyzed for weaknesses. This approach enables you to separate Tesamorelin fact from fiction, regardless of how widely a claim has circulated.

In Practice: Going From Myth to Evidence

Suppose you encounter a claim like, "Tesamorelin rapidly melts belly fat for anyone looking to slim down." The claim should prompt the following response:

- Write down the entire claim and where you saw it.
- Ask: Is there a scientific citation? Is it the result of a press release, testimonial, or retailer?
- If cited, does the referenced research involve general population weight loss, or only HIV-associated lipodystrophy patients?
- How long did any reported benefit actually take? Was it measured by imaging, physical exam, or simply patient self-report?
- Are safety risks discussed or downplayed?
- Is there an official regulatory or guideline backing for the context used?

If you cannot confidently follow the marketing claim to a robust, population-appropriate clinical study or approval, and if the claim omits or ignores side effects or approval status, it is likely hype or misinformation.

Tesamorelin's position at the intersection of medicine and wellness marketing means hype is prevalent and myths easily perpetuated. However, with a critical ruleset—flagging unsourced language, checking the true context for study findings, and tracing claims to their origins in authoritative literature—you can reliably bust common myths and dissect exaggeration or ambiguity. This not only protects against unwise decisions but fosters confidence in the value of evidence-based, personalized, and ethical Tesamorelin evaluation. By internalizing these principles, you root every conclusion about Tesamorelin in sound skepticism and verified science.

Interpretation Tools: Results, Statistics, and Practical Significance

Reading Tesamorelin research can be daunting: you'll be met with charts, graphs, percentages, and heavily-footnoted endpoints, all framed in clinical jargon. Yet, beyond the numbers, your goal is to make sense of both the reliability of the data and its actual meaning in a real-world context. This chapter sharpens your ability to interpret Tesamorelin study results using robust, skepticism-driven tools. Understanding these key principles will help you recognize when a claim is supported by meaningful evidence—and when it is simply statistically adorned noise.

Table of Key Statistical Terms and Thresholds from Tesamorelin Studies

Every rigorous Tesamorelin study is structured around precise statistical concepts designed to determine whether the treatment is truly effective, safe, or both. To anchor your reading and critical thinking, here is a table explaining the most commonly encountered terms and standards in published Tesamorelin clinical trials and regulatory reviews.

Table 10: Table of Key Statistical Terms

Statistical Term	Tesamorelin Context & Typical Thresholds
p-value	Assesses whether differences in outcomes (e.g., VAT reduction) are likely due to chance. A p-value < 0.05 is conventionally considered statistically significant in Tesamorelin research.
Confidence Interval (CI)	Displays the range within which the true effect (e.g., mean fat loss) probably lies, often reported as 95% CI. Narrower intervals suggest more precise estimates.
Endpoint	The primary result measured in a study, most often visceral adipose tissue (VAT) reduction for Tesamorelin.
Absolute Risk Reduction (ARR)	Occasionally used to quantify decrease in risk (e.g., new-onset diabetes), calculated as the difference in event rates between treated and control groups.
Relative Risk (RR)	Ratio comparing risk of an outcome (like hyperglycemia) in Tesamorelin users versus controls; RR above 1 means higher risk in the treated group.
Number Needed to Treat (NNT)	Tells how many patients need Tesamorelin for one to benefit in the prescribed endpoint, such as significant VAT reduction.
Adverse Event (AE) Rate	Proportion of subjects experiencing side effects, categorized by frequency and severity, and compared versus control/placebo.
Baseline and Change from Baseline	Indicates starting measurements (e.g., initial VAT) and the amount/percentage changed by the

	end of the study period—key in reading time-based Tesamorelin outcomes.
Treatment Duration	For Tesamorelin, typical studies last 12 to 26 weeks—understanding this influences both the relevance and expectations of clinical significance.

Recognizing these terms and their thresholds allows you to quickly assess whether a Tesamorelin trial result is strong, marginal, or weak in its evidence.

Checklist for Distinguishing Statistical from Real-World Significance

A classic misunderstanding occurs when statistically significant findings are confused with meaningful, practical, or real-world benefits. It's vital for any Tesamorelin evaluation to separate these two domains especially because a drug may show impressive numerical changes in trials, yet offer little perceptible improvement for patients.

Use this checklist whenever you read a new result about Tesamorelin:

1. ***Is the difference statistically significant (usually $p < 0.05$), and how big is the observed effect in absolute terms?*** For example, if the study reports a mean VAT reduction of 10%, is that enough to matter clinically, or is it just a small shift made to look important by a large sample size?

2. ***Are the measured endpoints (like VAT reduction on CT scan) translated into real health outcomes, such as improved metabolic health or quality of life?*** For Tesamorelin, endpoints often focus on imaging-based fat measurements, with less frequent linkage to hard outcomes like reduced diabetes risk or better daily functioning.
3. ***How do the confidence intervals look?*** If a reduction in fat mass is reported with a wide confidence interval (e.g., –14% to –2%), the effect is less certain than if it's narrow (e.g., –6% to –4%).
4. ***Does the duration match patient needs and product claims?*** Most documented benefits of Tesamorelin require at least 12–26 weeks to appear, and rapid changes are unlikely.
5. ***Are common side effects or risks downplayed relative to benefits?*** For example, reductions in VAT might coincide with increased glucose intolerance, which can offset practical health gain.
6. ***Does the stated benefit apply to the same population and context as in your area of interest?*** Efficacy in HIV lipodystrophy does not automatically equate to general effectiveness for non-HIV populations.

By answering these questions, you can determine if the result is not only statistically measurable but also likely to have tangible value day to day.

Framework for Spotting Cherry-Picking, Overgeneralization, and Selective Reporting

Interpretation pitfalls aren't just about misunderstanding numbers; they're also about how data is presented—or withheld. Tesamorelin literature and marketing are not immune to the three most common distortions: cherry-picking, overgeneralization, and selective reporting.

Here's a framework to guard against each while reading Tesamorelin claims:

1. **Cherry-Picking:**
    - Look for whether positive endpoints (e.g., maximal VAT loss) are highlighted while neutral or negative ones (like insulin resistance or lack of muscle gain) are omitted.
    - Assess whether sample characteristics are especially narrow or selected to maximize effect sizes Tesamorelin studies that exclude anyone outside the HIV lipodystrophy population but later generalize to "everyone" are classic examples.
2. **Overgeneralization:**
    - Beware when findings limited to specific populations (such as those with HIV or metabolic syndrome) are presented as broadly applicable.

- Make sure the context of benefit (e.g., type of fat reduced, time required) matches the population in question. Just because Tesamorelin reduced VAT in clinical trial subjects does not guarantee similar effects in non-trial, overweight adults.

3. **Selective Reporting:**
   - Scrutinize whether all endpoints outlined in the study protocol are discussed in the findings, or only those that reached statistical significance.
   - Check supplementary data for unreported side effects or subgroups with poor results.
   - Be cautious with studies reporting interim analyses or subgroup only findings, which may exaggerate overall impacts.

Always cross-check original sources (like regulatory documents or fulltext studies) over summarized or headline-driven accounts, and ask: What is being left out, and would knowledge of it change the claim?

Template for Cross-Comparing Study Results for Consistent Patterns

Isolated studies, even robust ones, can mislead if their findings are not replicated or at least echoed in the broader body of evidence. Building a side-by-side comparison of

Tesamorelin outcomes from various studies sharpens your ability to spot genuine signals amid statistical noise.

Here is a basic template you can use to cross-compare Tesamorelin study results:

1. **Study Details:**

   Title/Source, Population (e.g., HIV lipodystrophy, general obesity), and Sample Size.

2. **Duration and Protocol:**

   Treatment duration (weeks/months), dosage, and measurement intervals.

3. **Primary and Secondary Endpoints:**

   E.g., VAT reduction, glucose metabolism changes, quality of life metrics.

4. **Statistical Results:**

   Absolute change, p-values, and confidence intervals for main outcomes.

5. **Side Effect Profile:**

   Frequency/severity of adverse events, with particular focus on metabolic disturbances or injection site reactions.

6. **Limitations or Caveats:**

   Was the study blinded? Was there a high dropout rate? Was the follow-up period sufficient?

7. **Real-World Translation:**

   Did the study report improvements that would be felt outside the clinic (such as energy, daily functioning, or ability to maintain weight loss post-treatment)?

Using this grid, circle or highlight patterns. For Tesamorelin, you might observe that most high-quality studies in the target group (HIV lipodystrophy) show moderate VAT reduction by imaging, but less consistent evidence of metabolic risk reduction or improved subjective well-being.

If you see one outlier study claiming extraordinary results or no side effects, weigh it against the averages and variances reported across the other data sources. Consistent replication strengthens the overall evidence for a Tesamorelin claim; isolated positive (or negative) findings warrant further skepticism.

Guide for Recognizing Insufficient or Missing Data and Reporting Limitations

A sophisticated interpretation of Tesamorelin evidence hinges not just on what's reported, but on what's missing or under-explained. Here are concrete ways to spot gaps:

- ***Short Study Durations***: If most outcome measurements cluster around 12–26 weeks, we lack clarity on long-term safety or sustained benefit yet, many marketing claims ignore this and imply enduring effects.
- ***Small or Unrepresentative Samples***: Studies with narrow, highly-selected samples (such as only males, or only those without comorbidities) lower the generalizability of any finding.
- ***Incomplete Adverse Event Reporting***: High-quality clinical studies and FDA reviews summarize all common, uncommon, and serious adverse events. If you see vague "no side effects" claims or missing numbers, the reporting is insufficient.
- ***Dropout or Non-Adherence Rates***: Failure to discuss how many participants failed to complete treatment or deviated from protocol makes for data that cannot be reliably applied outside the research setting.
- ***Lack of Comparator Groups***: Claims about Tesamorelin effectiveness without reference to placebo or active comparators do not indicate how much of the observed effect is due to the peptide itself versus expectation, natural history, or other interventions.
- ***Surrogate Endpoints***: Many Tesamorelin studies use changes in a single lab value or imaging metric instead of meaningful health outcomes. This should always be

disclosed and recognized as a limitation unless the surrogate is conclusively linked to hard health benefits.

- ***Absence of Postmarketing Data***: If a product has been on the market for years, but only pre-approval clinical trial data is referenced, ask why unreported postmarketing experiences may contain crucial information about rare or long-term complications.

Practical tips for noticing insufficient data:

- Scan the methods and results sections of studies for red-flag phrases: "Data not shown," "results available upon request," "interim analysis," or "no statistical difference noted."
- Look for transparency in side effect tables. Are both common and serious risks reported in numbers, not just as rare/none?
- Pay close attention to studies sponsored or prepped for marketing: are results shared in full, with negative or neutral outcomes included?

By staying alert to these limitations, you can avoid making decisions or recommendations based on incomplete Tesamorelin evidence, ensuring your assessment remains tethered to reality and away from wishful interpretation.

Interpreting Tesamorelin research with rigor requires more than reading an abstract or trusting reported outcomes at face value. It means mastering key statistical terms and thresholds, distinguishing between changes that are simply "statistically significant" and those that matter in real-world health or quality of life, and recognizing the subtle ways in which data can be misrepresented—through cherry-picking, overgeneralization, or selective omission.

Building comparative tables allows you to see patterns that isolated numbers may conceal, and a critical eye toward missing data or reporting limitations keeps you from succumbing to misleadingly optimistic summaries. With these interpretation tools, you are well-prepared to critically evaluate any new Tesamorelin claim, separating meaningful progress from statistical sleight-of-hand. These skills empower genuine, evidence-based decision-making in the ever-evolving world of Tesamorelin research.

Building a Custom Tesamorelin Evaluation Table

As you navigate through the flood of information on Tesamorelin, its precise uses, hoped-for benefits, and potential downsides you'll find that synthesizing it into a form that makes sense for your own decision-making is essential.

A structured evaluation table helps keep skepticism well targeted: it forces you to itemize claims, anchor them to their sources and evidence quality, and spot where uncertainties or trade-offs loom largest. In this chapter, you'll be guided step by step through the process of building, maintaining, and interpreting your own Tesamorelin evaluation table.

Step-by-Step Instructions: Assembling Your Personal Summary Table

Creating your Tesamorelin evaluation table is best approached as an iterative process, one that supports clear thinking now and remains robust for updates as new data or guidelines emerge. Here's how to get started:

1. ***Identify and List Key Claims***: Begin by reading clinical reviews, regulatory documentation, or scientific articles on Tesamorelin. For each promise, risk, or uncertainty you encounter such as "Tesamorelin reduces visceral adipose tissue" or "May cause glucose intolerance" start a new row in your table. Limit each claim to a clear, single-issue statement for easier tracking and assessment.
2. ***Link Every Claim to a Source***: Next, enter the specific source for each claim, being as granular as possible. As you list a benefit or risk, directly associate it with its supporting study, product monograph, or regulatory document, noting both the document and any evidence tier (e.g., randomized controlled trial, observational study, regulatory review). Clearly noting the strength and nature of the backing evidence is vital for differentiating robust findings from speculation.
3. ***Capture Measurable Outcomes***: For each efficacy or harm claim, include how the outcome was pragmatically measured. This might be a reduction in VAT on a CT scan, change in fasting glucose levels, or the incidence rate of an adverse effect like injection site discomfort. If the claim is vague or based on subjective measures, flag it for closer scrutiny.
4. ***Document Known Risks and Side Effects***: In a dedicated column, summarize the risk profile that has been directly linked with Tesamorelin in clinical

review reports and regulatory guidance. For example, common documented risks include joint pain, muscle aches, injection site reactions, and metabolic effects such as increased blood sugar or diabetes risk. Reference the clinical review for detailed listings where possible.

5. ***Register Outstanding Questions or Unresolved Uncertainties***: Not all evidence is conclusive clinical documentation often notes areas where more research, longer-term safety data, or larger samples are needed. Create a column to capture open questions or knowledge gaps, such as "Impact on cardiovascular events still unknown" or "No long-term real-world safety data in non-HIV populations".
6. ***Systematically List Practical Alternatives***: Where relevant, add a column for alternative approaches or comparator treatments. For example, if the benefit is "VAT reduction," note what other drugs, lifestyle interventions, or standard-of-care options are available, and whether they have been validated with stronger or equivalent evidence.

Essential Column Template for Maximum Clarity

Here's a template for the columns in your Tesamorelin evaluation table:

- Claim (concise, one-issue statement)
- Evidence Source (reference and tier/ranking)

- Measurable Outcome (how was the effect or risk assessed?)
- Known Risk (severity/frequency; as specific as possible)
- Open Questions (uncertainties, gaps in knowledge)
- Alternatives (treatment or strategy options with supporting references)

Each of these columns supports the goal of comparing and contrasting practical benefits and trade-offs, rather than making blanket yes/no judgments.

Example Entry (for orientation):

Table 11: Essential Column Template

Claim	Evidence Source (Tier)	Measurable Outcome	Known Risk	Open Questions	Alternatives
Reduces VAT in HIV lipodystrophy	FDA Review (RCT, Tier 1)	CT-verified VAT reduction	Hyperglycemia, injection site rxn	Effect after treatment cessation?	Diet, exercise, metformin
May cause glucose intolerance	FDA Review (RCT, Tier 1)	Fasting blood glucose, HbA1c	Same as claim	Frequency in non-HIV populations?	Lifestyle modification
Start working within 8-12 weeks	Expert Review (Clinical)	Imaging results, clinical charting	None specific, but ongoing therapy	Duration of benefit with continued use?	–
Injection site discomfort is common	Product monograph (Tier 2)	AE reporting in trial summary	Local pain/redness	Rate/ frequency over long-term?	Alternate administration

Rules for Periodic Updates

The landscape of Tesamorelin research is dynamic: new trials, postmarketing studies, or updated guidelines will appear, often making older conclusions less reliable. To keep your table accurate and aligned with best evidence:

- ***Schedule Reviews***: Set a calendar reminder to revisit your Tesamorelin evaluation table every 6–12 months, or after any significant regulatory, clinical, or marketing update.
- ***Update with New Evidence***: If a new study adds clarity on long-term Tesamorelin outcomes, or a new risk emerges from postmarketing safety data, add a new row or update the relevant claim, keeping older rows for transparency but flagging them as superseded where needed.
- ***Record Changes in Guideline Recommendations***: If professional societies issue guidance that affects the clinical use or safety profile of Tesamorelin, ensure your evidence source column reflects this and revisit all claims likely to be affected.
- ***Document Your Rationale for Changes***: Whenever you add, remove, or revise a claim, summarize why. Was it due to new evidence, a retracted study, or a change in regulatory language? This audit trail strengthens your own transparency and future-proofing.

Checklist for Consistent Terminology and Definitions

A common pitfall when aggregating information from diverse Tesamorelin sources is the inconsistent use of terms what's called an "adverse event" in one paper may be split into "serious" and "mild" adverse effects elsewhere; "lipodystrophy" may have different thresholds across documents.

<u>To guard against confusion:</u>

- ☐ ***Standardize Key Terms***: When you encounter a new term such as "VAT reduction", "injection site reaction", or "sustained response" extract how it is defined and ensure you use this definition throughout your table. If definitions vary from source to source, footnote those differences for later review.
- ☐ ***Be Precise With Clinical Criteria***: Whenever a study uses a formal outcome (e.g., "significant VAT reduction: ≥10% decrease by CT imaging"), record the numerical threshold or diagnostic tool used. This avoids conflating loosely defined claims with rigorous ones.
- ☐ ***Align Population Description***: If one study limits itself to HIV-infected individuals with documented lipodystrophy, label this population precisely in your evidence source column. Make it clear when a claim is

about a special subgroup, not the general adult population.

- ☐ ***Use a Glossary***: As your table grows, build a mini-glossary for recurring abbreviations and clinical endpoints (e.g., VAT, AE, NNT), tied to their source definitions. This supports comparison and helps other readers interpret your table unambiguously.

Protocol for Synthesizing High-Level Takeaways From Your Table

Once your Tesamorelin evaluation table is populated, it becomes more than just a passive record: it's a platform for deriving clear-sighted conclusions and actionable advice. To extract high-level takeaways:

1. ***Scan for Efficacy–Risk Balance***: Are the best-supported claims about Tesamorelin (e.g., VAT reduction in HIV lipodystrophy) paired with well-characterized, manageable risks, or are key questions about long-term safety left unanswered? Summarize the net balance for each indication, noting where benefits are robust and where uncertainty predominates.
2. ***Flag Areas of Strong or Weak Evidence***: Compare the evidence tiers across entries: which claims are anchored in randomized controlled trials with regulatory review, and which rest on single case

reports or open-label studies? Use color-coding or plain-text notes to show at a glance where evidence strength clusters and where skepticism should be highest.

3. ***Note Unresolved Questions***: Are there major open questions repeated across multiple sources—such as "insufficient long-term data," "unknowns in non-HIV populations," or "not compared to best alternative therapy"? Highlight these, as they point to the need for continued caution or additional research before broader adoption.
4. ***Distill Practical Decision Points***: For each major clinical or personal decision you might face—such as whether to recommend Tesamorelin to a particular patient group, or whether to pursue it as part of a wellness program—annotate your table with a summary of the balance of benefit, risk, and unknowns tailored to that scenario (without venturing outside established evidence or clinical recommendations).
5. ***Monitor for Shifts Over Time***: With periodic table reviews, track how patterns in Tesamorelin evidence and risk have shifted. Are original uncertainties closing with new trials, or are new concerns appearing? Recognize that your synthesized positions should evolve alongside the evidence base.

Additional Tips for Optimizing Your Evaluation Process

- ***Focus on Documented Start Times and Durations***: Evidence shows most measurable effects of Tesamorelin, such as VAT reduction, emerge after 8–12 weeks, not immediately. Ensure your "measurable outcome" and "claim" columns reflect realistic start times and avoid over-interpreting early anecdotal responses.
- ***Rigorously Separate Efficacy and Safety***: Don't merge benefit claims (e.g., fat reduction) with risk or side effect entries. Keeping them discrete enables clear-headed trade-off analysis—especially since adverse events like injection site pain or changes in glucose tolerance are often as important as the efficacy endpoints.
- ***Regularly Validate with Authoritative Sources***: Whenever possible, prioritize entries from FDA labeling, peer-reviewed meta-analyses, and clinical review reports for claims and definitions—resist the temptation to elevate marketing summaries or "testimonial" evidence above established scientific consensus.
- ***Treat "No Evidence" as Its Own Category***: If a commonly cited claim or concern about Tesamorelin (for example, anti-aging effects in healthy individuals) lacks any credible data, log this explicitly as "no evidence" in the relevant column. This distinction is

crucial for discouraging over-interpretation and pseudo-scientific adoption.

Your custom Tesamorelin evaluation table is much more than a tidy spreadsheet—it's your personal filter for hype, anecdote, and half-truth, driven by transparent, evidence-based reasoning. By rigorously listing claims, sources, measurable outcomes, risks, uncertainties, and comparators, you transform scattered research and conflicting commentary into a framework that supports clear, ongoing judgment.

With regular reviews and disciplined updates, your table will remain a relevant, powerful resource as Tesamorelin research and clinical practice evolve. This method doesn't guarantee certainty on every question, but it does ensure that your conclusions about both the potential and the limitations of Tesamorelin are grounded, justified, and as immune to trend-driven misdirection as possible.

Conclusion

Arriving at an informed conclusion about Tesamorelin means synthesizing the considerable evidence regarding its benefits, risks, and limitations. After applying the tools and frameworks outlined in the previous chapters, you are equipped to cut through marketing noise and anecdotal claims to make judgments grounded in evidence.

Tesamorelin stands out as a prescription medication specifically approved for reducing excess abdominal fat in HIV-infected patients with lipodystrophy. Its efficacy and safety are anchored in regulatory reviews and well-structured clinical trials. When used in line with approved indications, Tesamorelin can produce measurable reductions in visceral adipose tissue, usually starting to manifest within 8 to 12 weeks of consistent administration.

Clinical results demonstrate these effects using objective outcomes such as imaging, which adds credibility to claims about benefit. The foundational strength of Tesamorelin's claims rests most securely on those populations and endpoints directly studied during regulatory approval, particularly HIV-associated central fat accumulation.

Yet even in these best-supported scenarios, Tesamorelin's profile is not free from caveats. Its adverse effects are well characterized: joint pain, muscle discomfort, and injection site reactions are among the more frequent side effects, while metabolic disturbances like increased blood sugar or potential new-onset diabetes require additional vigilance, particularly in at-risk individuals.

Not all patients will experience the same degree of benefit, and the persistence of effect following discontinuation remains an area of unresolved inquiry. Additionally, long-term safety data, especially for off-label or non-HIV-related uses, are currently limited or absent, underscoring the importance of a cautious approach when extrapolating beyond studied populations.

One persistent risk in the Tesamorelin landscape is the overextension of legitimate findings. Marketing and secondary sources may imply applications or benefits not substantiated by strong data. For instance, claims about Tesamorelin's utility for anti-aging, general obesity, or athletic enhancement lack the backing of rigorous clinical trials and therefore should be flagged as speculative or unsupported. Being diligent in tracing each assertion back to its primary evidence source and rating the strength of that evidence using the table-building methods described previously guards against adopting unproven or potentially unsafe practices.

Making an informed decision means recognizing trade-offs. For candidates who meet established criteria, the expected benefits of fat reduction must be weighed against both common side effects and uncertainties about longer-term outcomes. Periodic reevaluation, prompted by emerging research or updated regulatory guidance, is essential for ensuring that one's assessment of Tesamorelin remains current.

Practical synthesis involves more than cataloging data points; it involves making peace with what is currently unknown while vigilantly monitoring for new evidence. By relying on transparent sourcing, standardized definitions, and clear separation of efficacy and risk, your evaluation table can act as a decision aid that is robust against hype and anchored in clinical reality.

In summary, an evidence-based approach to Tesamorelin is not about seeking certainty, but about approaching each claim, benefit, and risk with proportional skepticism and clarity. When your evaluation process is methodical, regularly updated, and honest about limitations, you are well placed to navigate Tesamorelin decisions with confidence and integrity whatever new information may arise.

FAQs

Why is Tesamorelin prescribed?

Tesamorelin is an FDA-approved medication specifically indicated for reducing excess abdominal fat in people with HIV-associated lipodystrophy. Its use is supported by clinical evidence and regulatory approval for this targeted population. For other uses, including general obesity or non-HIV-related conditions, Tesamorelin is not recommended.

How does Tesamorelin compare to other growth hormone–releasing agents?

Tesamorelin differs from other growth hormone–releasing agents due to its molecular specificity, unique approved indication, and clinical usage profile. Unlike direct growth hormone analogs, Tesamorelin stimulates the body's natural growth hormone release by mimicking GHRH, leading to a more physiological hormone pattern. It is currently the only GHRH analog approved for treating excess visceral fat in HIV-infected individuals with lipodystrophy, while other agents lack such approval or robust clinical backing for this use.

Clinical trials have thoroughly evaluated Tesamorelin's risk–benefit profile for this specific population, whereas other peptides or GH secretagogues remain mostly experimental or off-label. In contrast, direct GH analogs can carry higher risks of adverse effects due to unregulated hormone exposure, whereas Tesamorelin's feedback-mediated mechanism may limit such risks.

What evidence supports Tesamorelin's long-term safety profile?

Tesamorelin's long-term safety has been chiefly evaluated through clinical trials and post-marketing surveillance in adults with HIV-associated lipodystrophy. It is generally well tolerated, with common side effects including injection-site reactions, joint pain, muscle aches, and sometimes transient increases in blood sugar or insulin resistance.

While some patients have shown minor increases in fasting glucose or developed diabetes especially those with pre-existing metabolic risk, major safety concerns have not emerged in studies up to one year. Ongoing real-world monitoring is essential, as rare or long-term effects might only appear with wider use. Proper patient selection and regular monitoring help minimize risks, and regulatory agencies continuously review new safety data.

Are off-label or anti-aging uses of Tesamorelin supported by high-quality studies?

Currently, there is little robust evidence supporting off-label or anti-aging uses of Tesamorelin. Most research has focused on its intended use for HIV-associated lipodystrophy, with few studies in healthy older adults or the general obese population.

No large, randomized trials have shown clear anti-aging benefits or improved body composition in populations outside those with HIV-associated fat redistribution. Claims found on wellness or anti-aging platforms are often based on theory or anecdote, not solid clinical evidence. Due to this lack of data, regulatory prescriptions and insurance coverage typically do not support off-label use.

How can one verify that a claim about Tesamorelin is credible?

To verify claims about Tesamorelin, check if the source cites reputable, peer-reviewed publications, regulatory agencies, or primary clinical studies. Look for evidence from well-designed clinical trials, consistency with guidelines from medical authorities, and transparency in reporting study methods and results. Be cautious with claims lacking clear references or relying on testimonials or marketing language. Always check if the information is current and reflects the latest research, including post-marketing data.

Can modifications of dose or administration method change Tesamorelin's risk–benefit trade-off?

Tesamorelin's safety and effectiveness depend on following the approved dosing regimen (typically once-daily subcutaneous injections). Changing the dose, frequency, or method of administration may increase the risk of side effects or reduce efficacy. Overdosing can raise the risk of adverse effects like glucose intolerance and fluid retention, while underdosing may make the treatment ineffective. Any changes to dose or administration should only be made under the guidance of a healthcare professional and based on clinical evidence.

References and Helpful Links

Carr, A., Samaras, K., Burton, S. et al.. (1998). A syndrome of peripheral lipodystrophy, hyperlipidaemia and insulin resistance in patients receiving HIV protease inhibitors. https://doi.org/10.1097/00002030-199807000-00003

Stanley, T., Feldpausch, M., Oh, J. et al.. (2014). Effect of Tesamorelin on Visceral Fat and Liver Fat in HIV-Infected Patients With Abdominal Fat Accumulation. JAMA. https://doi.org/10.1001/jama.2014.8334

Smaila, B., Holland, S., Babaeijandaghi, F. et al.. (2020). Systemic hypoxia mimicry enhances axonal regeneration and functional recovery following peripheral nerve injury. Experimental Neurology. https://doi.org/10.1016/j.expneurol.2020.113436

Ishida, J., Saitoh, M., Ebner, N. et al.. (2020). Growth hormone secretagogues: history, mechanism of action, and clinical development. JCSM Rapid Communications. https://doi.org/10.1002/rco2.9

Wang, Y., Tomlinson, B.. (2009). Tesamorelin, a human growth hormone releasing factor analogue. Expert Opinion on Investigational Drugs. https://doi.org/10.1517/13543780802707658

Bedimo, R.. (2011). Growth hormone and tesamorelin in the management of HIV-associated lipodystrophy. HIV/AIDS - Research and Palliative Care. https://doi.org/10.2147/hiv.s14561

Falutz, J., Potvin, D., Mamputu, J. et al.. (2010). Effects of Tesamorelin, a Growth Hormone–Releasing Factor, in HIV-Infected Patients With Abdominal Fat Accumulation: A Randomized Placebo-Controlled Trial With a Safety Extension. https://doi.org/10.1097/qai.0b013e3181cbdaff

Cicione, A., Nacchia, A., Guercio, A. et al.. (2023). Cardiovascular adverse events-related to GnRH agonists and GnRH antagonists: analysis of real-life data from Eudra-Vigilance and Food and Drug Administration databases entries. Prostate Cancer and Prostatic Diseases. https://doi.org/10.1038/s41391-022-00640-4

Sattler, F.. (2013). Growth hormone in the aging male. Best Practice & Research Clinical Endocrinology & Metabolism. https://doi.org/10.1016/j.beem.2013.05.003

www.ingramcontent.com/pod-product-compliance
Lightning Source LLC
LaVergne TN
LVHW022006200926
848481LV00007B/2259
* 9 7 9 8 3 4 9 3 1 1 5 6 7 *